How to write a scientific paper

—

advice from the editor

JACOB ROSENBERG

Copyright © 2016 Jacob Rosenberg
All rights reserved.
1st edition.
ISBN-13: 978-1535337434
ISBN-10: 1535337435

ULTIMATE RESEARCHER'S GUIDE SERIES

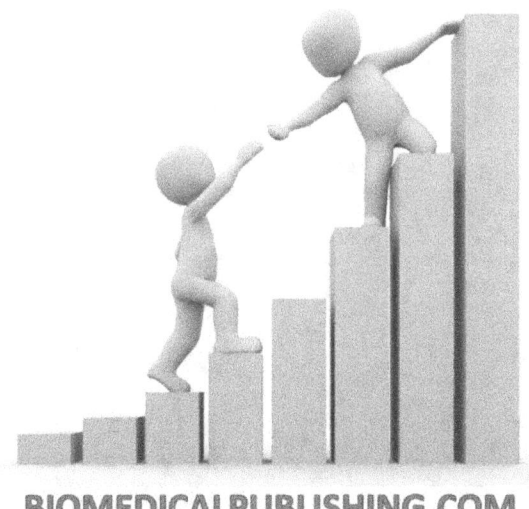

CONTENTS

PREFACE **6**

INTRODUCTION **9**

PART 1: SECTIONS IN A SCIENTIFIC ARTICLE **12**
- *A good title for your paper* *12*
- *How to write an abstract* *15*
- *How to write an introduction section* *20*
- *How to write a methods section* *23*
- *How to write a results section* *26*
- *How to write a discussion section* *30*
- *How to use tables and figures* *37*
- *Your image is in the reference list* *42*

PART 2: BUILDING OF THE ARTICLE **49**
- *How to build an original article* *49*
- *How to build a protocol article* *60*
- *How to build a systematic review* *64*
- *How to build a narrative review* *72*
- *How to build a case report* *76*
- *How to build an editorial* *80*

PART 3: STYLE TIPS AND CLOSING REMARKS **83**
- *A few style tips for medical writing* *83*
- *Closing* *94*

NOTES **95**

CONTACT **97**

PREFACE

This is the first in a series of books where I will guide you through various aspects of the writing process for scientific papers and how to get them published. In the present book I will go through the different sections of a scientific paper and discuss how to build it paragraph by paragraph. The key to success is to use the same technique every time you write a paper, because then the writing process will be much easier for you. You don't have to invent the wheel every time you write a paper, so stick to a pre-defined detailed outline and the end product as well as the writing process itself will be much better.

I have headed a research group for a number of years. This research group belongs to a large public university hospital and we have over the years developed a special technique for writing scientific papers. It is very effective in that it can almost cure writer's block, and it makes the production of at least three papers per year per research assistant possible and at the same time preserves the technical quality of the papers. I will of course also teach you this technique in one of the upcoming books.

Thus, the main purpose of this book series is to help you overcome the learning process as fast as possible in order to facilitate your development into not only a top researcher but definitely also to a top scientific writer.

There are numerous problems that you may encounter doing research and writing papers and my goal is to give you tips and tricks so that you can overcome some of the most common problems that you may encounter. Of course I cannot write the papers for you, but I hope that you will get some tools in your toolbox so that you can get your papers written and published without it being a really big workload for you. For sure, there are many issues that I am not covering, so if you have a specific wish for something I should cover in a future new edition of this book or in another book, then you are more than welcome to write to me. Please use the contact form at the home page www.biomedicalpublishing.com and I will do my very best to include it in a future book release.

Enjoy!

Introduction

I have been editor of two medical journals for a number of years and also served on the International Committee of Medical Journal Editors (ICMJE) for seven years and thereby have a profound interest in biomedical publishing. The ICMJE is also called the Vancouver group and it consists of 12-14 personal members that are elected every time a seat becomes vacant. Typically, the ICMJE consists of members from the so-called big journals and also from smaller journals and from different parts of the world. It has been fantastic to work on this committee for the seven years, and I have really learned a lot.

In my job as editor I have seen a lot of mistakes and terrible writing, but of course also a lot of brilliant papers. One thing that seems to be obvious is that papers that follow a distinct pattern or outline usually are easier to read. And remember - this is probably the most important thing that we should focus on both as writers and as editors. The papers have to be fairly easy to read because otherwise the reader will leave you immediately and move on to other material that they can digest without a great work effort. This is certainly the trend nowadays where there are way too many papers published for the individual researcher to read. Therefore, you have to make the reading experience pleasant and interesting. And there are definitely writing tricks to use here.

One of the most important hints for scientific writing is to use the same template and technique every time you write a paper. That is why the present book will cover exactly that – to use a strict template for every scientific paper that you write, This will make things a lot easier for you, because as soon as you are familiar with the writing process using the same technique every time, then you can much better focus on what you are actually writing, i.e. you will then be able to improve the content quality of the paper at a much faster pace. Think - if you would be struggling with the writing technique for many years, then your own personal development as a science writer would be severely postponed. Therefore, it is important that you as fast as possible learn the technical aspects of scientific writing, and thereby you will much faster be able to write really good papers to be published in top journals.

> *"One of the most important hints is to use the same template and technique every time"*

The book is divided in 3 parts. Part 1 will go through the different sections (title, abstract, introduction, methods, results, discussion, tables and figures, references) of a scientific article. Part 2 will take you through the actual building of the different article types (original article, protocol article, systematic review, narrative review, case report, editorial), and part 3 will give some selected style tips and closing remarks.

Part 1: Sections in a scientific article

A GOOD TITLE FOR YOUR PAPER

It may be a challenge to choose a title for your paper. Sometimes you will give it a very dull and boring title and in other cases the title may be too long. Often authors can experience that the editors have actually changed the title of their scientific article. This is because the titles typically in submitted manuscripts are either bland or too cryptic for the readers. There are a few tips when it comes to naming your article and it is fairly easy to follow these.

First of all it is a good rule to remember that the title should not ask a question but rather provide the answer. There should preferably be no question marks, no exclamation marks, no citations, percentages etc. There should also not be names of geographic locations or years in the title unless it is very important for the message, and finally the title should include a verb to make the sentence active.

"The title should not ask a question but rather provide the answer"

An example could be an article that may originally be called "Is a hernia a hereditary disease?". Instead the article should be called "Hernia is a hereditary disease". In this way the reader is not irritated by the question and instead he or she will get the answer immediately. This is much better and therefore please avoid question marks in the title. Another example could be for instance a title such as "Death at hospital X in children with disease X in the years X and X". That can be activated by changing it for example to "Number of deaths in children with disease X is increasing". In this way you avoid the name of the hospital and also avoid the years, and the sentence has become active by the verb. The title will make the reader interested and it gives the answer rather than raises a question.

Of course there are exceptions to these rules, for instance if you want to write a paper on the outbreak of bird flu in a special province in China or something like that, then of course it will be relevant to include the name of that geographic place in China in the title and also the year, but in almost all other cases I will say that you should avoid places and time, and make the title active with a verb and give the final answer to the research question. These are effective ways to make the reader interested.

Another situation is that some journals prefer that you put a colon after your title and then include the study design, for instance "Hernia should be repaired with a mesh: a

"You can place a colon after your title and then include the study design"

systematic review". It is actually a good idea to do this, but mostly for systematic reviews and meta-analyses, and also for randomized controlled trials, because then the reader will immediately see in the title that this paper is of high quality and then again - the reader may be more willing to read your paper, and this is actually what it is all about. So, it may be a good idea to put the study design after the colon if the editors will allow that, especially for papers of higher evidence levels.

In conclusion, the title should be short, active, give the answer rather than pose the question, and it may be a good idea to include the study design after a colon. The overall purpose of title is very simple - you can use it to attract the readers to your paper. It will be digested very fast and you have to get the readers interested and invite them inside. You have to get them interested so that they will actually read your paper and not continue their search and their browsing for other papers that are out there. There is so much available literature nowadays and so many papers are coming out each day so you really have to think carefully about the title. The title is your tool to attract readers.

"The title is your tool to attract readers"

How to write an abstract

In the previous chapter we discussed how to give it a good and inviting title and now you have to look at the abstract. The title as well as the abstract are actually two of the most important parts of the paper because they will sell the message to the editor and in the next round to the external reviewers, and if the article is published it will also be the title as well as the abstract that will make sure to invite the reader inside, and then your paper will more frequently be read. So, please spend time producing a good abstract because it is extremely important for your paper.

Very often when people write scientific papers, then they spend a lot of time writing especially the discussion section, but actually you should spend much more time on the abstract because it is the abstract that is the really important part of the paper. It will appear on PubMed and other search engines and this will actually be the thing that most readers will read and some of them will not even read more than the abstract. So spend a lot of time writing a good abstract – it pays off in the end.

"The abstract is very important"

The abstract should be written in a way that it could stand alone. That means, that it can be read without the readers have to read the full article. There is therefore no reference to information in the paper itself and it's obviously very important to adhere to the journal's limits for lengths of the abstract. This is typically around 200-300 words, but check the author guidelines because they will say exactly how to write the abstract, if it has to be structured or it has to be narrative and the accepted length of the abstract.

The writing style of the abstract is typically a little more telegraphic than in the rest of the article text, because you simply don't have the space to produce long and nice sentences. If possible - and this is actually quite important - avoid using abbreviations and avoid the passive form. Use active form instead and as in the rest of the article text you should use short sentences and relatively simple language. Avoid an over-academic language that will scare the readers away. This is actually a ground rule for all academic writing that you should use simple language but still with precise medical phrases of course. Don't make it too academic and with strange words and complicated sentences because that will make it more difficult to read, and also more difficult to write.

If the journal wants a structured abstract, which is the most common form, it will typically be divided into background or introduction, methods, results and conclusion. Sometimes the journal

"The structured abstract is the most common form"

will ask for a specific paragraph with the study aim, but that is not always the case.

So in this first background section you should tell the reader briefly what is known previously in this area and why the current study is needed, and then you specify the purpose of the study or aim of study.

The next will be the methods section or the methodology section depending on the journal again. In this section you should tell very briefly what you have done. This must be kept very short because details can be read in the article itself.

The next part will be the results. This section of the abstract is probably the most important section and you should start with the most important findings, the most important things first and then the secondary outcome parameters later. This results section should start by answering the research question and it should not only indicate the p-values, but also tell the reader about the magnitude of the fact. This can be done in different ways, but it is a good idea to include parameters such as medians and ranges for the different methods and then the p-values in a parenthesis.

> "The results section of the abstract is probably the most important section"

The magnitude of effect can also be shown in other ways of course and you should use the journal's traditions for this, for instance if they want 95% confidence intervals instead of p-values. So check the author guidelines and also read some previous articles in this specific journal and simply do what others have done here.

The abstract does not have a discussion section so the next paragraph will be the conclusion. The conclusion section of the abstract will provide the interpretation and the perspectives of the findings so this is also an extremely important part of the entire paper and of course the most important part of the abstract.

"The abstract has no discussion section"

Now, when you have written the full abstract you should do a little test, and that is to read the abstract without reading the paper and then you should ask yourself: So what? If this can raise some questions, if you need more information in the abstract, it is simply just to fill it in. So remember to do this final test. You can also do the test in people that have not actually read the abstract or the paper, which is of course much more powerful. So either yourself or others should read the abstract in the entire length and ask yourself if something is missing, then you can fill that in.

In conclusion, the title as well as well as the abstract are the most important parts of your paper and they will serve as the first entrance to the article, both for the editor and the peer reviewers and then finally of course for the readers when it is published.

How to write an introduction section

Now we will write the introduction section. This section can actually be written at a much earlier stage because you have all the necessary information from the research protocol but most often you will write the introduction section typically when you write your full paper.

The introduction section is important because this is where you will lose a lot of readers if you don't do it correctly. The typical error is to make the introduction section too long with too much information and this is just so wrong. In the introduction section you will have to make a firm grip on the reader, so that they will stay and read the rest of the article and it will also set the stage, so that the reader will understand what it is all about. If the introduction section is too extensive, then you will lose readers that will simply move on to other sources of information, which of course are abundant. So, you have to make it short and to the point.

> *"A typical error is to make the introduction section too long"*

A very good advice is to build the introduction section only with two text paragraphs. The first paragraph will set the stage for the clinical problem and briefly explain the lack of evidence in the area - but very short, maybe 12-16 lines of text or something like that. The second paragraph will briefly present the aim of study or the purpose of the study with or without the hypothesis behind it. Thus, the first paragraph will typically be 12-16 lines of text and the second paragraph only around 3 lines of text.

It is a good idea not to have too many citations in the introduction section. The purpose here is not to make a systematic review. The purpose is just to set the stage for the reader, so that he or she will stay and read the rest of the paper. If your paper has a long introduction section the classic scenario is that part of the text here can actually be moved to the discussion section instead. It is not intended that the introduction should describe in detail the entire subject area or justify the choice of your experimental design. Things like that belong to the discussion section. So, if you have a too long introduction section, then look at it in the way that you may be able to move some text to the discussion instead.

"Use only few citations in the introduction section"

There may of course be some papers where it is justified to have maybe three paragraphs in the introduction section, two background paragraphs and then the third will give the aim of study, but try to keep it short and try as often as possible to use only two paragraphs, one with the background, and one with the aim of study. This will keep the reader on board so he or she will move on and read the rest of the paper.

How to write a methods section

There are very few rules for the methods section. The two most important rules are first of all to try to write it in the chronological order. This means to describe the study methods in the order that you actually did it during the study data collection period. The second rule is that the last paragraph will typically include the study registration if relevant (e.g. www.clinicaltrials.gov or a similar registry) and permissions from ethical committees and so on, and then the statistical tests that you have used. So, it should be fairly easy for you to write your methods section.

"Permissions and statistics in the last paragraph"

If it has been a very difficult trial, then it may be a good idea to use sub-headings dividing the methods section into sub-sections, but in most methods sections I will say that this is not at all necessary and it can be written just as plain text with the normal division into paragraphs.

As mentioned it is typical to specify registrations, permissions and statistical methods in the last paragraph in the methods section. Some journals, however, they want this information in the beginning of the methods section, so you should check again the instructions for authors and simply do what they tell you to do.

If you have previously performed similar experiments, then you may be using the same sentences in this paper as you have written in your own previous papers, and this is actually plagiarism. It sounds crazy because it is your own text, but it is called self-plagiarism, and this is not OK because typically the text is actually owned by the publisher and not by you even though you wrote it originally, An exception to

"Beware of self-plagiarism"

this is if the original publication was in an open access journal where the publisher do not retain the copyright. So, be careful not to self-plagiarize yourself and do not copy-paste from your own previous papers. So instead of using the same sentences even though the methodology is the same, then you can simply refer to some of your previous papers where the methods have been described in detail.

Typically, the methods section is one of the easiest parts of the paper to write because you simply write what you did. It is not at all difficult and you can take your study protocol and then simply follow that and describe your research project in chronological details. Thus, if you experience the so-called writer's block, which means that it is difficult for you to sit down and write your paper, then a very good advice is actually to start with the methods section. This is called modular writing, and I will get back to that in much more detail in another book in this series. It is a way to write your paper not from the first to the last line, but to start with what's on the top of your mind. That could potentially be the methods section because it is easiest part of the paper to write. So, start with that if you have severe writer's block – that is a good advice.

How to Write a Results Section

The results section of a scientific article must explain what was found and nothing more - no interpretation of results - that's very important. The results section typically has no references and it only reports the study findings.

In most papers/research projects you typically will employ some kind of data reduction when you write your paper. It seems inappropriate, but nevertheless, typically in the design of the trial you have been too enthusiastic and you put too many parameters in. You may have wanted to gather data for this and that, and that is of course not a good idea. The optimal situation is that all data acquisition should be hypothesis-driven, but in daily research practice is it usual that researchers get a little over-enthusiastic and will collect more data than they actually need.

The best way to do it is to think everything through in the design phase of the trial, and actually at that stage make a detailed statistical analysis plan. Almost no academic researchers actually do that, but it is common practice in pharma-sponsored trials. That is the way to do it – to do a detailed statistical analysis plan at the time that you design your study because then you can see exactly what data you will have to collect in the

"Stick to your statistical analysis plan"

trial. So, do that – think it through – think about the final paper already in the design phase of the study. Then you will not do as much data reduction as you would otherwise typically do.

If you did not do a detailed statistical analysis plan in the design phase, then you will have too many data and you have to do some kind of data reduction. In this process it is of course not at all OK only to choose the positive findings, meaning the significant results and not the opposite. That is of course the wrong way to do it. You have to look at your primary and secondary outcomes and then you simply report those. All other findings are merely hypothesis generating, and you can choose to report some of them if they contribute to an interesting discussion and perspectives for future research. Regarding the findings around your primary and secondary outcomes, you will report these no matter their statistical significance. They have to be reported regardless of what you find, and needless to say that you of course have to stick to your definitions of primary and secondary outcomes from the initial trial design and registration. Thus, in the results section, you will report the findings that will support or reject the study hypothesis.

"Demographics in Table 1"

When you compose your results section you should always start with the most important findings first, and then state the less important findings afterwards. This means that you will start with study demographics because this will define your study material. This is typically given in detail in a Table 1. Then you go to the next paragraph and state the results concerning the primary outcome parameters. In the third paragraph (and maybe more paragraphs depending on how many secondary outcomes you have in your study) you give details for the secondary outcome parameters.

"Start with the most important findings"

It is a great idea to use tables and figures to supplement the presentation of your results. However, it is very important to use tables and figures only as an alternative to the text and not specify the same in both text and tables and figures. In your tables and figures you can give the details about your findings and in the text of your paper you will summarize it without p-values and without detailed numbers. For instance you will say "there were more men than women in the study" and then refer to the table. In the table you give the numbers (how many men and women) and if there was a significant difference (you state the p-value in the table). This is just a simple example, but in

"Details in text and figures and only a brief summary in the text"

general it is advisable to give details in text and figures and a brief text summary in the text in the result section.

The results section will present the results of your hypothesis to the reader. Start with the primary outcome and then followed by the secondary outcomes, and support your presentation with tables and figures. You can give detailed numbers and p-values in the tables, and then a brief text summary in the text in the results section. Figures can be used to show interesting trends and relationships between study groups, i.e. think of figures as a pedagogic tool to explain the meaning of the results to the reader. The journal will not like you to present 10 tables and 10 figures of course, but do it wisely and then the figures and tables will supplement the text and make it more readable and interesting.

How to write a discussion section

Traditionally, the discussion section of an article is considered to be the most difficult part to write, especially as a new author. However, there are some very good advices in the preparation phase, which can make it easier for you to write the discussion section.

Typically, for an original article, you should as a standard use six paragraphs in your discussion section.

The six paragraphs are these:

1) Basic findings
2) The primary outcomes
3) The secondary outcomes
4) Strengths and limitations
5) Perspectives
6) Conclusion

So, in the first paragraph you will state the basic findings or give a brief summary of the findings in the article. No numbers here, no p-values of course, because all these details are given in the results section. Just explain what the main findings were in your study as plain text. We normally say that you should tell it to the reader like you

"Basic findings in the first paragraph"

would tell it to a layperson like your grandmother. It has to be easily understood for everyone because many readers actually will read this first paragraph of the discussion section before they read any details of the study, so they will have to understand the essence of your findings without any prior knowledge of your study design or other study details. You may think that it is unnecessary to give the basic findings here since it will be a repetition of what was already stated in the results section, but it is a kind of service to the readers that they can jump to the first paragraph in the discussion section immediately and see what you actually found. The typical length of this first paragraph could be around 10 lines of text.

In the second paragraph you will discuss your primary outcome, and "discuss" means that you will include what other researchers have found and how do that compare with your own findings. You don't have to give a comprehensive systematic review including all other studies in the field, but you should put your own findings in perspective comparing your results with other similar studies. The typical length of this second paragraph could be around 10-20 lines of text.

"Primary outcome in the second paragraph"

In the third paragraph you will then discuss the secondary outcomes in the same manner as you discussed the primary outcome, meaning include previous studies and compare your findings to theirs. Remember to be a little bit humble when you discuss your secondary outcomes because your study was not designed to give robust answers regarding the secondary outcomes. The sample size calculation is always based on the primary outcome and therefore you cannot solve an important research question if it has only been a secondary outcome parameter in your study. There may be an exception here, if you actually powered your study to cover also the secondary outcomes but this is usually not the case. The typical length of this third paragraph could be around 10-20 lines of text.

"Secondary outcomes in the third paragraph"

The fourth paragraph will include strengths and limitations. It is a classical error only to mention your limitations. Why not also mention your strengths? You have done a great study and there is no reason to forget the strengths of the study. It is a good idea to start with your strengths and then give the study limitations after that. You have a choice what to include as your study limitations, because you can obviously not include all thinkable limitations in this text paragraph. All studies have

"Strengths and limitations in the fourth paragraph"

numerous limitations and potential sources of bias, and you should choose only the most important ones here. The typical length of this fourth paragraph could be around 10-15 lines of text.

The next paragraph, number 5, will include the perspectives of the study. This means you will have to briefly discuss the clinical importance of your findings. How do they convert to daily clinical practice? Remember to look at it with not only geographical local glasses on, but rather discuss the relevance of your findings in a global perspective. It is also in this paragraph that you will state if the provided evidence should be considered final or if more research is needed, and in this case what studies should be performed. The typical length of this fifth paragraph could be 5-10 lines of text.

"Perspectives in the fifth paragraph"

The final paragraph, the 6th paragraph, will be the overall conclusion of the study. It is common to begin this paragraph with "In conclusion, we found that..." or something like that. The essence is to clearly show the reader that this is the study conclusion paragraph, so therefore start with the words "In conclusion, ...". This last paragraph has to be

"Conclusions in the sixth paragraph"

short. The reader should be able to read it in only a few seconds, because many readers will jump right down to this paragraph before they read something else in the article and you therefore have to get them interested before they get tired and leave your paper for something else. Therefore, keep it short and to the point. No discussion here – our findings showed this and that and on one side it means this and on the other side it means that. No way. Discussions like that can be given in the perspectives paragraph. The last sentence in the conclusion paragraph will typically be something like further studies are needed – but alternatively you can have solved the mystery and thereby provide a final conclusion. This is unfortunately rare these days, as it typically would require very large patient materials. As a main rule, don't be overconfident in your conclusion but rather present your findings with a little bit of modesty here. The reader will judge the importance of your study by himself or herself. The typical length of this last paragraph of the discussion section could be 5-10 lines of text, but the shorter the better.

As a main rule for the discussion section it is extremely important not to present any results.

"No results in the discussion section"

They should be mentioned in the results section instead.

Most discussion sections can generally be reduced by maybe up to 50%, so be careful to make it brief. It is not the discussion section that is the most important part of your paper – it is actually the results section. Many authors feel that they have to sell their article to the reader by making a comprehensive and long discussion section, but it actually has the opposite effect. The reader will give up half way through the reading and leave the paper for something else. It is much more powerful to make it brief and to the point and thereby let the results speak for themselves.

"Keep it short"

Another typical problem will be if you use so-called "name-dropping". That should be avoided whenever possible. Name-dropping is if you for instance write "in previous work by Rosenberg et al. (ref), it was shown, that …". Instead you should write: "In previous work it was shown that… (ref)" and then the reference will take the reader to the paper in the reference list. It is called name-dropping when you write the name of the researcher in the text. This will disturb the reader a little bit, because, when the reader sees the name of the researcher in the sentence, then automatically the reader will try to think "do I know this guy?"– and it will stop the reading for a short moment, maybe only for some milliseconds, but it will slow down the reader. So don't use name-dropping and simply state what you want to say, and then give references to the previous papers.

"Avoid name-dropping"

So to summarize, the way to write a good discussion section is to make it very tight with only six well-defined paragraphs. Make it a habit to only use these six paragraphs – nor more and no less. This is a good habit when writing original articles. It is different for other article types such as a systematic review that only has 3 paragraphs in the discussion section, but an original article should have the same six paragraphs in the discussion section every time: 1) basic findings, 2) discussion of your primary outcome 3) discussion of secondary outcomes, 4) strengths and limitations, 5) perspectives, and 6) conclusion. Please make it brief and write in a reasonably simple language without too many different words, because the reader has to be able to read your discussion section without having to slow down and read your sentences all over again simply in order to understand them. Keep it brief and keep it simple.

How to use tables and figures

Use of tables and figures is an effective way to present the results of a scientific study and they can typically tell the reader much more than you can do with plain text. It is therefore a good idea to present the main findings of the study in tables and figures as the reader will typically look at the tables and figures before the text is actually read. This will invite the reader inside so to speak and the likelihood of the paper being read is much higher if you use tables and figures than if you don't.

It is important to take the time to make very educational and easy-to-read tables and figures, which should preferably be understood immediately by the reader. A typical error is when the figures are very complicated with double Y-axes or 3D effects or if they include too much information. If you have a lot of information then maybe split it into two figures instead of one. So please be sure to make them simple and easy to understand.

Tables and figures should not repeat information from the text but data from tables and figures can be exemplified in the text or be summarized in the text instead of in the tables and figures, where the data are much more detailed. This means for instance, that the

"Use tables and figures as an alternative to text"

numbers and p-values are given in tables and figures and the text will simply explain in simple language for the reader, what the results have shown, but without for instance mean values and p-values.

Most journals have an allowed maximum number of tables and figures and of course as an author you have to respect that. If you feel an urgent need to publish additional tables or additional figures you can ask the editor if you can provide those as for instance additional material available only on the web. This is done quite often nowadays, that the journals will put extra material along the pdf and html-file of the article, and this additional material will only be available in the web-version of the journal.

In the paper you will have to number the tables and figures chronologically in the order they appear. There is, however, an important thing to stress here, and that is that every table legend and figure legend is considered to be independent text passages. This means, that if you use an abbreviation in the main text and you also want to use it in the legend to a figure, you actually need to define that abbreviation all over again in every figure legend and every table legend even though you have defined it already in the main text. That is because every figure and every table

> *"Every table and figure legend is independent text passages"*

should be readable on its own without having to read the full paper.

Typically, table 1 is used for baseline characteristics of the patients and figure 1 is typically used for a flow chart of the participants in the study. This may of course vary depending on the study design and the journal, but this is the typical situation.

"Demographics in table 1 and study flow chart in figure 1"

Tables and figures should be inserted in the manuscript on a new page for each and they will appear after the list of references. Most journals will have a single page with legends to tables and figures and other journals will like to have the legends be put under or over each table or figure, but the typical situation is that they will require a separate page with all the legends together.

Most journals will want the figures in separate files uploaded in the electronic manuscript system, but you have to check the guide for authors for each journal. If they want for instance figures in separate files you will have to produce for the submission process a separate title page in one file, the main text including references in one file and then separate files for each figure and each table to be uploaded separately. But again – check the instructions for authors and then you will know exactly what to do. Then the question is: what kind of files do you produce for the figures? Tables should always be in Word-format or similar. Never submit a table as a spreadsheet file like Excel. You could save your figures as jpeg-files or similar, but most journals will actually like to have the original artwork, meaning that if you have made the file in for instance GraphPad or PowerPoint, then they often would like to have the original file, because then they also get the data actually, and if they want to redraw the figures, then they can do that now having the original data behind the figure. Other journals will like to have the picture file instead, for instance a jpg or png-file. So again, you have to check the instructions for authors before you submit anything.

When talking about legends for tables for instance, then some authors tend to give a table a heading that is put above the table and then some footnotes below the tables typically the abbreviations or something like that. However, the journals often do not like that. They want everything presented together so put everything in one single table legend and then let the journal decide how to handle it – that is the best solution.

Finally, you should know, that it is actually quite costly for journals to publish tables and figures, as they will require work from a graphics designer to put it into the special journal layout. Therefore, consider carefully if all your individual tables and figures are really necessary for the paper - if they will significantly increase the value of the article to the reader. For instance, if you want to put a large table in a systematic review and this table will include all the evaluated articles, then you should know that such a table is often only of marginal value to the reader and actually it is mostly only of value for you as an author to retain an overview of the data in the writing process. So maybe you should skip this large table in the manuscript itself. Alternatively, you could put it as an additional file only on the Internet version of your article, because if you do that, then most journals will not put it in the special graphics design of the journal and they will allow this file to be a simple text file without special journal formatting. So this could be a good solution, and you could then in the text just refer to the table as an additional file in the web-version of your article.

> *"Large tables can be published as supplementary files"*

In summary, use tables and figures because it will increase the readability of your paper for the reader, but you have to make them quite simple and they have to be necessary, meaning that you can put specific data in tables and figures and then you in the main text can just summarize what you have shown in detail in the tables and figures. This will make it easier to read the main text and the very interested reader can go to tables and figures and find the detailed data there. Do not make it too difficult to read and if you want to present very large tables you may be able to do that as additional files only on the web-version of your paper.

Your image is in the reference list

In this chapter I will discuss something that seems to be a continuing problem. That is to avoid errors in the reference list. Try to look at it from the editor's point of view. If you as an editor receive a paper where there are numerous errors in the reference list what feelings would that produce? I mean simple errors like wrong use of commas and colons or wrong abbreviations of the journal names. Editors are humans and it will create a negative feeling in the editor's mind and it will actually raise a suspicion of other errors as well. If the author cannot do a proper reference list, then maybe the study itself is also full of flaws errors. So, your actual image as a researcher is reflected in your reference list! Therefore, please focus on that and never ever again submit a paper with errors in the reference list.

"Avoid errors in the reference list"

It is really important to stress that there are always errors in the reference list if you only rely on your reference management software. You have to remove the codes from the reference list and go through it manually word for word and look at everything in detail before you

"Reference software often makes errors"

submit the article to a journal. Everything has to be checked in detail and all errors corrected.

So what should you do in detail? You should first of all go to the journal's website, the journal where you want to submit your paper, and then look at previous articles in your target journal and look at how the references are printed, because you should do your references in exactly the same manner. Also of course you should double-check the instructions to authors and look for detailed guidance there. And you really have to do this in a serious manner. Don't skip anything and go through your references one by one.

> "Go through your references one by one"

Typically, the journal will want the names of the authors with the surname first and then initials for the given name divided by commas between the authors. Then a full stop followed by the title of the article that you are referring to. Then often the problems start because the abbreviations of journal names sometimes will tease you a little bit. However, there are some easy tricks here, because you can look in PubMed for help. If you go to the PubMed webpage at pubmed.com then on the right side of the screen, there is a link to "Journals in NCBI Databases". If you press this link then you can write the journal name or just part of the name in the search bar. Then the journal name and abbreviations and many more details will come up and now you have the correct abbreviation of the journal name. After the journal abbreviations in the reference list, then typically, but there are some variations here, the year of publication will come and then a semicolon and then the volume number and a colon followed by the page numbers. Typically the issue number will not be given in the list of references but only the volume number. Then there are some variations also in whether you should put a full stop after the last word of the journal abbreviation name. That differs from journal to journal. So look it up in detail and of course do as all the other papers have done in that particular journal.

"Journal abbreviations can be found on PubMed"

There is a typical question that arises when you want to cite a paper that has not been published yet. The overall rule is that a paper that has only been submitted for publication and is not yet accepted cannot be cited as a reference in the reference list. So if you have a paper that is only submitted you can either wait and submit your own article later when the reference paper has been accepted, or you can put it in the text instead and call it "personal communication" in parentheses. If the paper has been accepted for publication you can easily put it in your reference list and typically you will just state the author names, the title, the year and a colon or a comma and then state "in press". That is the normal way to do it. If the paper has been so called pre-published as "e-pub ahead of print", then you can provide the DOI-code after the journal title because that will refer the reader exactly to the e-pub version of the paper before it has been assigned to a specific volume and with page numbers in that specific journal. But again, go to the Instructions for Authors and that will tell you exactly how to refer to papers that have been accepted for publication but have not yet been published.

Another typical question is whether you should cite the primary publication or if it is OK to cite a later review article summarizing many previous references in the area. The overall rule is of course to go back to the original reference and cite that. It may be OK to cite a more recent review paper instead if your target journal has limitations on how many references you are allowed to use in your current paper. For instance if your current paper can only have maybe 30 references, then it may be difficult to cite all the original articles with the original sources and then it may be OK to cite a few review papers instead. If it is possible you should always cite the original work and not a later article.

"Cite the original publication"

It is often stated that self-citations are bad and that you should limit that to an absolute minimum. The understanding that use of self-citations is only done to boost your personal number of citations, i.e. your H-index, probably drives this opinion. There may be some truth in this of course, but sometimes the use of self-citations is a natural and correct way to cover the specific research field if your studies are central. Thus, there may be areas where you have actually done most of the research and in that case there are no other ways than to cite your own work.

A typical problem in the reference list is when you are citing other things than papers in scientific journals, for instance when citing books, web pages, social media, or newspapers. When you cite books it is really important to look in the instructions for authors and in the reference list of other papers because when citing books there are many variations. Normally you of course will give the author name and if it is a book that has been edited by other authors then also the editor's name for that particular book, and thereafter comes the book title. Typically, you will of course give the year of publication but also the publisher's name and the city where the book was printed, and then of course the page numbers. However, as mentioned above there are many variations for this, so look in the "Instructions for authors" and get guidance there.

When you want to cite Internet pages the best way in my opinion is to use one of the archiving options on the Internet, for instance www.archive.org, but there are many of these around so you don't have to go to this particular one. Choose one of them and it is quite easy to log in to those sites, create a web-archive for your specific web-page that you want to refer to, and then you will now refer to the web-archive URL instead of the original URL. This will secure that the particular web page will be available forever and not only for a short period of time, because web pages will typically change. That is why an internet-reference will be short-lived if you do not use an Internet archive as reference instead of the actual Internet web page URL.

> *"Use archiving options on the Internet"*

If you want to refer to social media it is actually the same problem as with Internet web pages because these references will be short-lived if you don't use one of the archiving options. You can take a snapshot of the social media web page and save it in a web archive and then you can refer to that because it will then be saved forever. If you want to refer to something on Facebook then this information will change within a few hours and the URL will then be totally different. So, it is a good idea to save that information in an archive and then use that as a reference instead.

There are challenges when talking about the reference list and the most important message I want to give you is that you have to take responsibility. You have to go through it meticulously, you have to go through every single reference manually and correct all the different errors that will be there, because reference management software still makes lots of errors.

Part 2: Building of the article

HOW TO BUILD AN ORIGINAL ARTICLE

In this chapter I will show you how to actually build your original article. In previous chapters you have seen the contents of the different sections and their paragraphs, but now you will have to put it all together to a full scientific paper for publication.

Depending on your work habit you may control the writing process in different ways. No matter how you work on a manuscript I would strongly suggest that you first of all make a detailed outline, and thereafter write the different paragraphs and sections. In another book in this series I will show you different ways of handling this process, but as soon as you have your outline you will compose your original article exactly the same way every time you write a paper. Do it always exactly the same way - no difference. This is maybe the most important message from me to you - to keep it simple - so choose a working method that actually works for you and never do something different, because then it is very easy, and you don't have to think about all these practical things. You simply now have to fill in all the blanks in the outline expanding the language to a full paper. This makes it very easy for you to write your scientific article.

Most electronic manuscript systems that are used for upload of the paper require that you prepare a set of files instead of one single document containing everything. Thus, typically they will want separate files for title page, abstract, body of the paper including references and tables, but the figures will be in separate files for each figure.

> *"Electronic submission often requires separate files for title page, abstract, main text, and each figure"*

I would, however, suggest that when you write your paper you put everything in one single Word document. Then it will be much also easier for your co-authors to make suggestions for changes and do critical revision if they only have to handle one single file. After all the authors have revised the manuscript, you can depending on the journal split the file and submit the number of separate files that they want for upload. The actual build of your original paper is like this:

First of all you will have to create a title page. The title page should of course consist of the title of the paper, sometimes, depending on the journal, they will also want a short running title, but that is not always the case. You can check the instructions for authors to see if they want that.

After the title you put the byline and that means the names of the authors who fulfill the ICMJE authorship criteria (www.icmje.org). After the authors you will give the affiliations meaning which departments and which hospitals the work originates from. After that you will give the name of the corresponding author, and that is typically the name of the first author, but that is not always the case. It can be anyone in the byline, but typically it will be the first author. In older days the contact information was almost exclusively by normal snail-mail on paper so at that time we put here the physical address of the corresponding author, but nowadays everything is by e-mail, so you only state the name and email address of the corresponding author. Then it is routine also to put a short statement if reprints will be available - this is also a little old-fashioned nowadays but especially if it is a commercial research study where a pharmaceutical company afterwards would like to buy reprints to give out to potential customers/clinicians, then it should be mentioned here if reprints will be available, or if they will not be available.

The next page is typically the page containing the abstract of the paper. On the top of the page you will put "Abstract", and then depending on the journal there will be, most typically, some subheadings because structured abstracts are becoming much more common than the narrative abstracts, so the typical abstract for an original paper will contain for instance: Introduction, Methods, Results, and Conclusion. Some journals want other subheadings so check the instruction for authors and divide the abstract into the correct subheadings. This was page number 2 containing the abstract.

On page number 3 the actual paper will begin, of course beginning with the introduction section. Most journals want a headline named "Introduction" but a few journals will just want the text for the introduction section without a heading. So again, check the instruction for authors on how to do it here on the top of page 3. As mentioned in part 1 of this book, the best way to build your introduction section, is to try to keep it as short as possible and to the point, meaning one paragraph with background and one paragraph with aim of study – nothing more. Only if it is very complicated you may put maybe two background paragraphs and then the aim of study, meaning three paragraphs in total, but try to keep it only in two paragraphs because that will make it much easier for the reader and will attract more readers to move on and read the rest of your paper. So introduction sections should most often be quite short, absolutely not more than one page in Word format with double-spacing.

The next section of your original paper is the methods section. There are no strict rules on length here because that of course depends on what study you have done. Typically, the start of the methods section will somehow define your cohort meaning your patient group or animals and how you collected the data, and then further down the line in the methods section you will have descriptions of all the things you did in the study. The only quite fixed rule here is that typically in the last paragraph we put the statistical tests used in the study and also all the permissions obtained as well as the study registrations. So for instance you will say data were described with means and standard deviations if

"Randomized trials are reported according to the CONSORT statement"

they followed a normal distribution and otherwise with a non-parametric method approach with medians and ranges for descriptive purposes and the two groups were compared with e.g. the Mann-Whitney test for those kind of data and other tests for other kinds of data, and then you will say that $p<0.05$ was considered statistically significant and the data were also given with their 95% confidence intervals if appropriate an so on. So, it depends on how you have chosen to describe your data and which statistical methods you have employed in your article. After this - but in the same paragraph - you will put all the permissions. This could include "The study was approved by the Local Ethics Committee" and then give the approval number and it was approved by a mandatory data protection agency or similar depending on local regulations of course. If your study for some reason was exempt from ethical committee approval it is important that you state that explicitly with an explanation. All these approvals are put here in the last paragraph of the methods section.

Finally, you will also here put the registration information because all trials have to be registered in a public database before inclusion of the first patient. That is very important because all these registrations are time logged, so afterwards everybody can see what date you actually did the registration and also what date the first patient was included. So please be careful here and register your study before inclusion of the first patient. There are many different registries at the moment (about 20) around the World and it really doesn't matter where you register your study. I personally would recommend clinicaltrials.gov because this is the largest registry, they are quite professional in handling of the information and it is free of charge. So I would recommend that. It takes maybe 30 minutes or so to register your study and then you have complied with all the rules. So back to the paper, you will write that the study was registered at clinicaltrials.gov and then give the registration number in parenthesis. All together the methods section will typically consist of maybe 4-7 paragraphs, but it depends on the study design of course.

The next section will be results and the composition of the results section also of course depends on your study. However, there are some ground rules you can use which will make it much easier for you to write and also for the reader to read the paper. The normal way to compose your results section would be first to give the demographics of your study cohort. This means, that the first paragraph will describe how many patients you have included and how they were distributed between different variables, e.g. how many men and women etc. Here it is typical to refer to table 1 and table 1 will give the demographics of the study cohort. The next paragraph of the results section will deal with your primary outcome parameter whatever that is and again, here it is a good idea to put the details in a table or maybe also a graph, but at least in a table, and refer to that. That was the second paragraph of the results section that was your primary outcome parameter. The third paragraph of the results section would then deal with the other outcome parameters, the secondary outcomes. You may have several secondary outcomes, but if possible put them all in the same paragraph - the third paragraph here in the results section. Again, use tables and figures if it will help the reader. The next one or two paragraphs will deal with whatever other findings you have come up with which will support or oppose your study hypothesis. To conclude here on the results section, there are no firm rules on how many paragraphs you have to include, but typically it ends up with maybe 4 or 5 paragraphs.

Then we move on to the discussion section and here there are some very good advices. Typically, the discussion section may be the part of the paper that you may think is the most difficult section to write, but that is absolutely wrong because the discussion section has some very strict rules for its composition and if you simply just follow those – then it becomes a piece of cake.

First paragraph of the discussion section will be something that we call "basic findings". In this paragraph which will typically be 5-6 lines of text you will explain in plain language with no numbers and no p-values your main findings. It should be described in a way that you can actually explain it to your grandmother, meaning a person with no specific knowledge about the research question. Explain it in plain English and simply tell the story. What is the most important story to tell from your study? This should be the first paragraph of the discussion section and we call it the basic findings.

The next paragraph will discuss your main outcome parameter. When I say discuss I mean that you should of course again very short state what you have found, again with words without numbers, because all the numbers are given in the results section and in the tables and figures. After stating what you have found, you will compare the findings with the literature. Thus, you say what you have found and then what others have found and why there may be a difference.

The third paragraph will discuss all your other outcome parameters, all your other results in one single paragraph, If it is an extremely complicated study you may here also do another paragraph, but preferably only basic findings in the first paragraph, the primary outcome parameter in the second paragraph and all the other outcomes in the third paragraph. Now you are actually done with the discussion of your own results comparing it with the literature.

The next paragraph is paragraph number four in the discussion section. This is what we call strengths and limitations. It is not only limitations, you are also very much allowed to put the strengths of your study because you have of course made a very good study and there is no need to only be negative. Start with the strengths, maybe using 5-6 lines, and then in the same paragraph go directly to the limitations. The limitations should probably cover around 6-8 lines.

Now we have come to the fifth paragraph in the discussion section and that is what we call perspectives. In this fifth paragraph you will try to look at your results from a helicopter perspective and look down on the entire globe and try to discuss the clinical impact of your results. What does it mean for future patients? Can we change patient-care based on your results?

Then finally in the sixth paragraph of the discussion section it is time for the conclusion. Most journals do not want a heading here saying "Conclusion". Instead it is normal routine just to start the sentence with the words: "In conclusion, …". Don't be too self-confident because there are of course potential flaws and biases in every study, so be humble but still underline what you have found.

After the conclusion it is time for a new page with all the literature references. They have to be numbered consecutively in most journals and be absolutely without any errors - so check the instructions for authors carefully how they want the references to be set-up because all journals are different unfortunately, and then you will make your reference list in the correct way.

After references it is typical to have the next page with legends to figures and tables. This means that the title and explanatory text for every figure and every table should be put in a page for itself, and after that every single figure comes on a new page and every single table comes on a new page.

This is everything – you are actually done now. Write the cover letter - submit it, and have a big party because you did a great job.

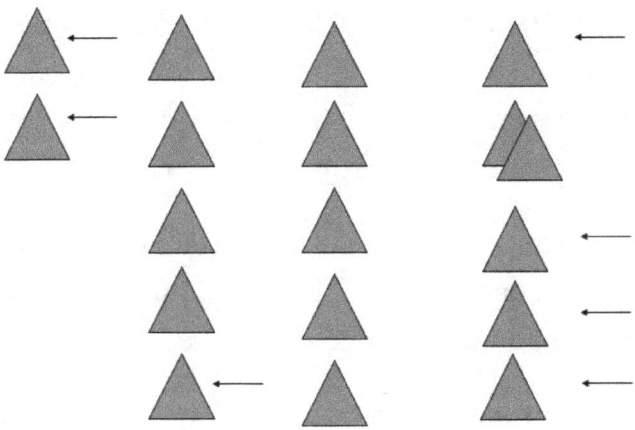

The figure shows the composition of an original article. Every triangle is a text paragraph and the arrows indicate pre-defined content:

Introduction: Background, aim

Methods: Statistics and permissions

Discussion: Basic findings, strengths and limitations, perspectives, conclusion

How to build a protocol article

A protocol article is a special kind of scientific paper where you will describe the design of your study and your statistical analysis plan. The statistical analysis plan is the most important part of the protocol article. The protocol article, because it is only describing the design before the study actually is running, will not have any results, so that makes the paper different from a normal original paper.

In the abstract you will give, as usual, the background or introduction and then the methods, but there is not a results section and then at the end there is a conclusion.

In the paper itself it will start with the introduction, which will, as usual for original papers, give first of all a paragraph with the background information, and then the second paragraph stating the aim of study.

Then there is a methods section and the methods section in a protocol article is of course the most important part of the paper. So that has to be quite extensive and actually often more extensive than the research protocol itself and certainly more extensive than the information that you have put on for instance www.clinicaltrials.gov because on that website and other similar registries you cannot give a lot of details about your methods. In the protocol article you have the opportunity to really go into depth about your methods. You will describe the primary and secondary outcome parameters, the sample size calculation, and the statistical analysis plan, which is the most important part of a protocol article. The statistical analysis plan has to be very detailed. You have to give information on exactly which variables you will test against which variables and you have to give the exact statistical methods. You will tell the reader how you will describe your results, and how you will perhaps build multivariate analyses models and so on. You should go into as much detail as possible and when you write your paper you will have to stick to this analysis plan. Therefore, think carefully since the analysis plan will bind you.

There is no results section, so the next section will be the discussion section. Usually this will be quite short and consist of few paragraphs, maybe 3 or 4 paragraphs at the most, where you will discuss the perspectives and the importance of this study, why it has to be done, and what it will add to the literature when you have your results of the study.

Now the text of the protocol article is finished. It will as always be a good idea to include tables and figures because it will be easier for the reader to actually read your paper if it has illustrations. You can choose whatever you want, but usually a study flow diagram will be good and maybe a simple table with inclusion and exclusion criteria. The choice is yours.

If you are doing a large clinical trial it is a very good idea to produce a protocol article and especially focus on the statistical analysis plan. That is actually the main reason for writing a protocol article. There are some journals, especially the most famous journals with high impact factors, they will publish your statistical analysis plan along with your original article if they accept your paper. However, most journals will not publish your statistical analysis plan and that is why it is a great idea to put that information in a protocol article before the first patient is included in your study. Then you have to stick to that plan afterwards when you do the data analysis and you cannot go on a fishing expedition in the data set. There are therefore many good reasons to do a protocol article, so don't hesitate - do it!

Protocol article

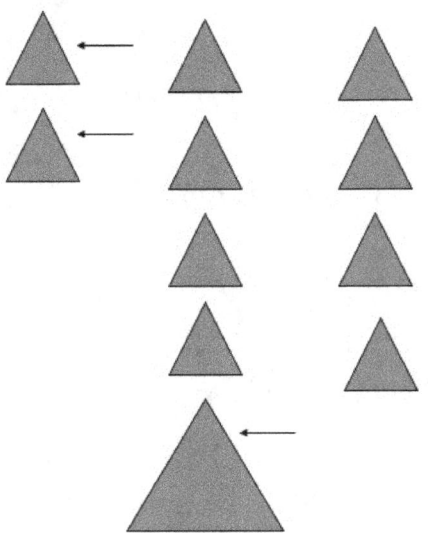

The figure shows the composition of an protocol article. Every triangle is a text paragraph and the arrows indicate pre-defined content:

Introduction: Background, aim

Methods: Statistical analysis plan (large because it is the most important part of the protocol article)

How to build a systematic review

You will see that there are many similarities between the build of an original article and a systematic review. That is because the systematic review is also presenting data, but here the data originate from other articles and not from a single patient cohort as in a standard original article. The building of a systematic review strictly follows the PRISMA guidelines (www.prisma-statement.org). The PRISMA guidelines will tell you how to report your systematic review and meta-analysis and it is very easy to follow. The checklist is so wisely made, that you can actually see how many text paragraphs your systematic review should be composed of and what exactly should be put in each paragraph.

"The building of a systematic review strictly follows the PRISMA guidelines"

The title is very important because this is the tool that you can use to invite the reader inside - to make the reader read your paper instead of just skipping it and move on to some other material on the Internet. That is why the title is important and you should really dedicate some energy here. A good advice for the title is that the title should give the answer instead of posing the research question. This means that for instance instead of saying "effect of anticoagulants after myocardial infarction" you should say "anticoagulants will reduce mortality after myocardial infarction: a systematic review". This is a really good advice that we have learned from the journalists that always put the answer upfront in the beginning and then after that they can elaborate in the main text of a newspaper article for instance. So give the answer upfront instead of posing the question. Another good advice for the title is to include a verb. This will make the sentence active instead of passive. You should not use question or exclamation marks in the title - only plain text and then it is easier for the reader to digest it quickly. According to the PRISMA guidelines, it is mandatory to put the words "a systematic review" or "a meta-analysis" after the title. This means that the title should be "anticoagulants will reduce mortality after myocardial infarction: a systematic review". Then the reader immediately can see that this is a systematic review and then it will more easily be found in electronic searches. It also has a psychological effect on the editor and the peer reviewers showing that this is a high-quality paper that they should look at with a positive mind.

Now we move on to the introduction section. This should preferably only consist of 2 paragraphs - this is also according to the PRISMA checklist. The first paragraph should describe the clinical problem and explain to the reader why there is lack of evidence. It means why it is relevant to do the systematic review. In the second paragraph you put the hypothesis and the aim of the paper.

Do not use to many references and a long introduction section will lose your readers so keep it short. Then it will move the reader further on down in the paper, so that your wise words will actually be read.

The next section is the method section and of course here it is very important to give the detailed search string for your literature search. Most often you give the search string for the PubMed search and then you can just write that this search string was modified to fit the other databases databases like EMBASE or whatever databases you have used for your literature search. The search string (including date of the search) will make your review reproducible which is a key factor for transparency in a systematic review. You should also in the methods section describe bias and confounding factors, you should describe how you have evaluated the quality of the papers, details about data extraction, and then also give information on the registration procedure of your systematic review. It is a very good advice to register your review at the PROSPERO database. You can just google PROSPERO and systematic review and University of York (because it is hosted by University of York in England) and then the link to the web page comes up. It is free of charge to register your review at PROSPERO. It is recommended but not yet mandatory to register the review because it will ensure that you have actually done what you intended to do and you have not made fishing expeditions during your data analysis. It will also help other potential authors of systematic reviews to see that they should not waste their time on exactly the same design as you have done and then they can do a slightly different design in their systematic review. This registration information should be put at the end of the methods section. You get a registration number from the database and this should be stated here at the end of the methods section.

The next section is the results section and again here you should follow exactly the PRISMA guidelines. In this section it is important to follow your protocol without any data reduction. This of course can only be done if you have really thought it through to begin with, the design of your study and especially which parameters you should extract from the papers. That is why you should really think very careful about your data extraction when you design your study. The clue here is to see the final paper in front of you, imaginary of course, and then you can see how you will build it, which tables you want to put in, which data will be relevant, and thereby you can extract only the data that you are actually going to use and thereby avoid data reduction. In the results section it is normal to refer to tables and figures and here you should not put the same information in the text as you put in the tables and figures. You should use tables and figures as an alternative to the text and not repeat the information. This means for instance that you can put the actual numbers and the statistical analyses in the tables or figures and then in the text you should just say with words that there were more men than women or whatever you find and then refer to the table, and not give the actual numbers and p-values in the text but leave that detailed information for the tables and figures. It is more convenient for the reader to have it this way and therefore it is a good idea because we always want to please the readers to keep them on board. Always when we write papers we want to please the readers by making it an interesting experience but still an easy task to read your paper.

The next section is the discussion section and here the PRISMA working group has really saved a lot of concern for the authors of systematic reviews. They have made this very simple because they explicitly only want three paragraphs in the discussion section. Normally, the discussion section is where the authors kind of show off. They want to show they are clever and true academics and they can compare their results with other studies, but this is not so important in a systematic review. So the discussion should be kept really short and very simple. Among editors we tend to say to each other that most discussion sections can be cut by 50% without any negative effects on the paper. Of course this is not always true, but it is a sign of many discussion sections being much too long. So keep it short and keep it simple.

The first paragraph in the discussion section will give the basic findings. This is a short summary of the main results only in words; no numbers and no p-values, just describe the main findings in plain language. When you write this paragraph you should think of things that you want to tell to a non-medical reader. In the second paragraph you will state the study limitations. This is e.g. the possible bias in the studies in the review. I do think actually, that you should elaborate a little more here and give both strengths and limitations because of course there are strengths in your study as well. So give both strengths and limitations in this second paragraph of the discussion section. In the third paragraph you give the conclusion of your paper but before you go to the actual conclusion you could use maybe 2 or 3 lines for the perspectives meaning what impact your findings may have on daily clinical practice. Thus, you can put perspectives and conclusion in one combined single paragraph in the end. This gives a total of only 3 paragraphs in the discussion section: 1) basic findings, 2) strengths and limitations, and 3) perspectives and conclusion.

In summary, the composition of your systematic review looks very much like an original article but the discussion section is shorter with only 3 paragraphs. The introduction and methods and results are comparable to the original article in their composition. In the introduction section you have two paragraphs, one is the background and two is the aim of study. In your methods section you give the detailed search string for PubMed and then supplement that with some wordings about how you changed it to fit the other databases. In the last paragraph in the methods section remember to put your registration number for the PROSPERO database. In the discussion section you only make 3 paragraphs. The first is basic findings, the second is strengths and limitations, and the third is perspectives in conclusion. The composition of the different sections in a systematic review follows strictly the PRISMA checklist so you can look there and see the exact information you have to include and how many paragraphs this will involve in each section of the paper.

Systematic reviews

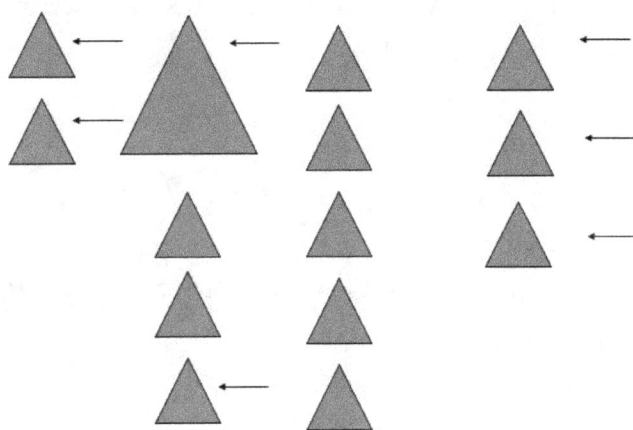

The figure shows the composition of a systematic review. Every triangle is a text paragraph and the arrows indicate pre-defined content:

Introduction: Background, aim

Methods: Search string, registration information

Discussion: Basic findings, strengths and limitations, perspectives and conclusion

How to build a narrative review

Nowadays, it is not so easy to publish a narrative review unless you are an opinion leader in the field. Some journals, especially the newer journals that are looking for content, will take narrative reviews also from less known authors, so if you have the time and energy to do it, it can be great fun. It is not always easy to write a narrative review because you have to know a lot about the clinical field or the area that you will write about. The reason is that there is no exact guideline on how to write a narrative review so you have to have some kind of an overview of the area in order to be able to write about it. This is an opposition to the systematic review, where there are very detailed guidelines from the PRISMA statement. In the narrative review, there are no specific guidelines.

"There os no guideline for a narrative review"

The introduction section should as always be kept short and to the point. Try to use only two paragraphs where the first paragraph will be the background and the second will be the aim. Don't use too many references; only enough to build your arguments for the review. The detailed review of the literature is saved for later text sections.

After the introduction section it becomes challenging because now there are the so-called "free topics". You can divide these sections into sub-sections or paragraphs just as you please and to whatever makes sense in the specific area that you will write about. You will typically have maybe four or five areas of interest in your narrative review and these areas should have a headline each.

After these free topics it is not always that you see a discussion section in a narrative review, but I personally think that it is a good idea because then you are allowed to put your text into some kind of perspective and you can discuss the area more freely. If you do a discussion section, which I would advise you to do, then divide it into paragraphs just as you are used to in other kinds of papers, meaning that the first paragraph in the discussion section will be some kind of a basic findings or overview of what you have just told the reader in all your free topics before that, and then maybe one or two paragraphs discussing your findings or your story in the free topic sections before the discussion section. The important part in the discussion will be the perspectives meaning that you should discuss what this actually means in clinical practice. What does it mean for the patient or for the health care provider or whatever topic you are writing about. The perspectives are very important. It is not normal to give strengths or limitations in a narrative review because there obviously are limitations in a narrative review and everybody knows that. And then of course as always, you should at the end give a conclusion where you can put it all together and try to give the overall statement for the reader in a very brief format.

If you have time and energy to write a narrative review it is great fun and it is a good idea, but it is a little bit more difficult than to write a systematic review, and may sometimes be a challenge to get it published. However, it will also teach you a lot about writing, so it is not a waste of time.

Narrative reviews

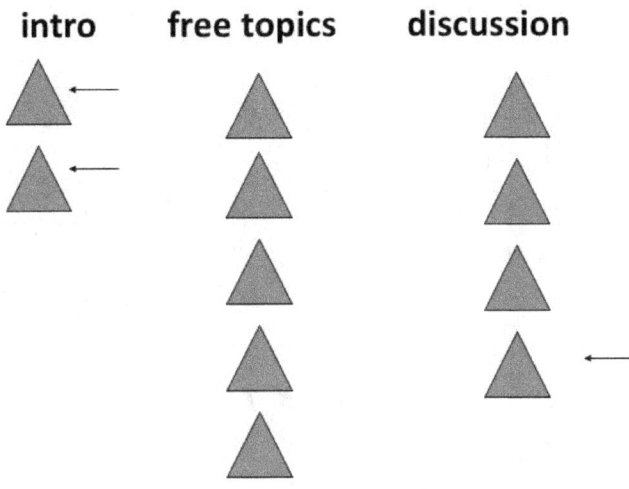

The figure shows the composition of a narrative review. Every triangle is a text paragraph and the arrows indicate pre-defined content:

Introduction: Background, aim

Discussion: Conclusion

How to build a case report

A case report is a quite simple scientific paper but of course it has to follow certain rules. There is a guideline published and you can find it on a website called www.care-statement.org, and it will guide you through the process of building your case report. There are some good advices for a case report and that is of course to keep it very short and then to focus on the learning points for the reader.

"The CARE statement will guide you to compose your case report"

According to the CARE statement the title of the case report should include the words "case report". The abstract is of course quite simple because you only typically have an introduction or background section, the case summary, and the conclusion.

The introduction section of the paper itself will consist of exactly the same as when we talked about building an original paper, it only has two paragraphs, the first being the background and the second will be the aim. In the CARE statement they recommend that you also produce a time-line for the case report. Personally, I find it to be a little bit difficult in practice, so if it makes sense to you, then do a time-line but if it does not make sense then you can perhaps skip it.

Then you will in the next section of the manuscript have the case story itself and that has of course to be divided into different sub-sections, not with their own head-lines but just text paragraphs consisting of e.g. the story, the physical exams, the diagnostic test results, what interventions were performed, follow-up, and outcomes.

After the case story you will go to the discussion section and a good advice would be in the first paragraph to give a kind of basic findings or the basic statement that you want to give the reader. State the exact learning points and underline the important issues. Don't hide it or make it a secret; explain exactly what you want the reader to take home. In the CARE statement they want strengths and limitations in the first paragraph, but I think that it is actually a little difficult to give strengths and limitations for a case report. Of course there are limitations for a case report. You cannot write a case report and then discuss how things could be for a total population, that's for sure, but it will have some learning points which will be important for the reader and that will always be the strengths of a case report. That is why I recommend you to put the learning points in the first paragraph of the discussion section because that will always be the strengths of a case report. The next paragraph will typically be some kind of a discussion, where you put your results or case story in relation to what has been published previously in the literature. Then you will again underline the learning points and may be if you can suggest a testable hypothesis based on your case. The last paragraph will give the conclusion and maybe perspectives for patient care.

You should always put some kind of illustrative material in a case report. That could be a picture, a CT-scan, a figure that you have produced yourself, or maybe a small table. It will make the paper a more interesting to read.

Now that you have written your case report the problem arises because you have to get it published and it is not always so easy nowadays to get a case report published in a scientific journal. However, there are some new journals out there that will only publish case reports. They are typically open access, meaning that you have to pay a fee to have the case report published.

Find an interesting case in your daily clinical practice and write a case report - it is fun and it is a reasonably easy paper to produce and then it will be good training for you also. It is also a good scientific paper to begin with if you are not a very experienced writer.

Case reports

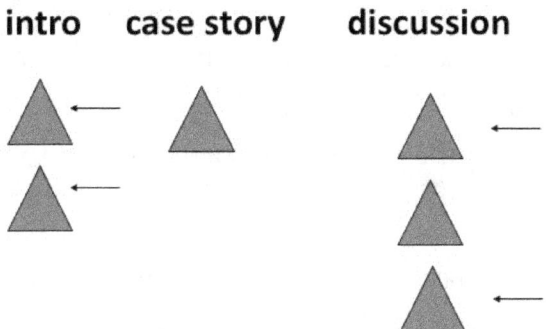

The figure shows the composition of a case report. Every triangle is a text paragraph and the arrows indicate pre-defined content:

Introduction: Background, aim

Discussion: Learning points, perspectives and conclusion

How to build an editorial

An editorial is of course not the first paper that you will produce in your academic career, but some day hopefully, you will be asked to write an editorial. It is great fun because it is kind of free play because you can almost write whatever you want and you can be very direct and even personal sometimes. You can hit somebody who needs to change their opinion, so it can be great fun to write an editorial.

There are basically two kinds of editorials, one being the paper written by the editor giving information from the journal to the reader regarding journal matters or editorial matters. The other kind of editorial is the one that you can write some day and they will typically be a kind of an opinion piece, but of course it has to be relevant to all readers because the editorials are generally read much more than the normal papers in the journal. An editorial is an important article in a journal and it has sometimes quite big impact actually, not impact as an impact factor because as you of course know, a single paper cannot have an impact factor - that is a journal thing to have an impact factor - but it has impact on maybe political decisions or other important issues in health care.

> *"An editorial is an opinion piece — short and to the point"*

When you write your editorial you should keep in mind that an editorial is a short piece. It can only be one printed page, sometimes two, so you have to keep it short. An editorial will usually not have any subheadings. Usually we say that an editorial is built like a fish. What does that mean? It means that you start with the nose and then you build it up. You make your arguments and build the content of the editorial, you expand and it gets bigger and bigger, covering the body of fish, which is the widest part. At the end you can give it a smack with the tail so to speak because you can say something honest to maybe politicians or other decision makers.

You start with a paragraph that will introduce the content of the editorial, why it is important. Then typically there will be maybe 4-6 paragraphs dealing with one specific issue in each paragraph. Don't mix things together because it will make it confusing for the reader. Keep it very concise and very strictly divided so one paragraph is only concerning one specific part of the problem. At the end you are allowed to really tell your opinion and maybe ask for change or whatever you want to say in your editorial.

An editorial is a really fun paper to write. You have to keep it very short and you only should write it if you really have something on your mind that you want to tell the readers. If you want to change something, then an editorial is exactly the right instrument to use.

Editorial

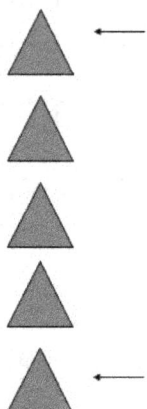

The figure shows the composition of an editorial. Every triangle is a text paragraph and the arrows indicate pre-defined content (see text for details).

Part 3: Style tips and closing remarks

A FEW STYLE TIPS FOR MEDICAL WRITING

In this chapter I will give you some selected style tips for medical writing. It is not intended to be a thorough grammar lesson but I will cover some of the most common and important problems that I have seen through the years, and they represent problems that are frequently encountered by novice as well as more experienced authors. From the editor's point of view these errors are annoying and why not please the editor? He or she will decide to accept or decline your paper. Most journals will send your manuscript to a copy editor for language and grammar correction before publication, but the reason to prevent these errors in the first place is not to avoid their publication but more to avoid irritating editor and reviewer, so that your chance of acceptance will be higher.

First of all, the wording "compared with" is used more often than "compared to". Why is that? When you speak English it is perhaps not so important to distinguish between compared with and compared to. Compared with is a bit softer in the pronunciation. Usually you use "compared with" if you compare something that is almost the same, whereas "compared to" is used when you compare something that is completely different. In medical writing it is most often the case that you compare something that is almost the same. You don't compare apples to oranges (different fruits), but maybe you compare two different patient samples (all human beings) and then you will use compared with. Thus, typically in biomedical papers you will use compared with.

What is the error: "Melatonin levels were higher in men compared to women"

(Should be "compared with")

The next point is when to use capital letters in scientific papers. When you describe drugs there is a difference between the name of the drug when you go to the pharmacy and ask for this specific drug or it's generic name. The trade name is always spelled with a capital letter as the first letter and the generic name is always spelled with small letters throughout the word. An example is the trade name Tylenol® and the generic name acetaminophen. Another example of using capital letters is kind of a new trend in medical writing and that is when you say for instance "on day 1 of experiment 2" then day and experiment is spelled with a starting capital letter. This is in fact not correct English as far as I know, but this is a trend in medical writing so "Day 1 of Experiment 2" is spelled with starting capital letters. Also when you put the words "table and figure" in your running text it is spelled with a capital T and capital F, for instance if you write "as shown in Table 2 and Figure 1", then the T and the F will be capitalized. You will never use capital letters in your references, also not if it is actually capitalized in the original reference when you see the article on paper or on the screen, but this should not go into your reference list.

What is the error:

"1. Pommergaard H-C, Andresen K. Effect of Intercourse on Mood Level in Healthy Volunteers. J Mood Physiol 2014; 23: 106-8."

(Capitals in the paper title words)

The next thing is when to use full stop and how to manage that. I know, that many schools are still teaching to put two spaces after a full stop in running text. However, this is not the case in scientific articles, where we use only one space after a full stop in the text. There are some exceptions where we do not use any space after full stop and that is at the inside of abbreviations for instance like e.g. or i.e. then you do not use a space after the inside full stop but only after the last full stop. If your sentence is ending with an abbreviation with a full stop, then of course you will not put another full stop after the abbreviation. If you are using abbreviations only with capital letters like for instance the NATO or USA, then there are no full stops.

What is the error: "Melatonin was highest at night. This was not the case in monkeys"

(Two spaces after full stop)

Another problem with spaces is when to put a space between a number and a unit, in formulas and before references. If you want to say 25 percent, then it should be 25% and not 25 %. Thus, there should be no space between the number and the percentage. If it is a result with a measuring unit, then you should give it a space between the number and the unit, e.g. 25 ml. Formulas always use spaces, i.e. a + b = c. If you give references in parentheses, then always use a space, i.e. "it was shown in a previous study (1)".

What is the error: "it was shown in a previous study(1)"

(a space is missing before the reference)

The next thing is about when and how to use a colon. If you use a colon in English medical writing, then there is not necessarily a capital letter after the colon. For instance you can say "Effect of sunburn on metabolism of alcohol: a systematic review" - then the letter "a" is not capitalized. Be careful when you use colon in the running text because it is a little difficult to do that and it will slow down the reader. The language becomes too difficult and it is better to rewrite the sentence without the colon. It is important to keep the language and sentence construction simple in order to make the reading experience fast and pleasurable for the reader, so my advice to you is to avoid using a colon in your running text of the article.

What is the error: "Effect of sunburn on metabolism of alcohol: A systematic review"

(should be small "a" after colon)

The next thing is the use of a semicolon. This is also a little difficult, but it can be used when you want to distinguish between different things, things that are truly different, for instance on one hand it is like this; on the other hand it is like this. You can also use it instead of a comma if you want to give the reader a longer pause when reading the text, for instance in a sentence like "the committee dealing with the question of commas agreed on a final text; however, the issue of semicolons was not considered". So, you can use it when you want to give the reader a longer reading pause in the middle of a longer sentence. However, as mentioned above about the use of a colon I would advise you to be cautious when using a semicolon and perhaps try to avoid it because it will make it a little more difficult for the reader to read your text and this is not our goal. Our goal is to make it easy to read and thereby actually also easy to write.

The next issue is use of a comma in the running text. I must say that the English use of a comma is very much different from the Danish use of a comma and I am a Dane, so it is probably quite difficult for many non-English authors to use comma correctly in English writing. The overall advice from me as a former editor would be to use comma not so often as you may be used to use it in your own language. If you are in doubt if there should be a comma in a sentence then better skip it than include it. Of course commas are used and especially when you want to give the reader a small pause when reading the sentence, then a comma would be in place. So, the general advice is to listen to the sentence and if there is a pause, then put a comma. Another situation where a comma is justified is when you are giving a list of different words divided by commas, for instance sugar, beef, milk, and butter. Another place where comma is normally used is after the small starting words in sentences, words like furthermore, moreover, however, in addition, in conclusion, and so on. These words are always followed by a comma because there is a small break. There is a small pause in the sentence, and this should be indicated by a comma. When using the word "respectively" at the end of a sentence there should also be a comma before that.

What is the error: "Sugar, beef, milk and butter"

(there should be a comma after milk)

What is the error: "Furthermore melatonin levels were higher in men compared with women"

(there should be a comma after "Furthermore")

The next thing is really irritating and that is the use of singular versus plural when writing your verbs in a sentence. Why is this so difficult? Many manuscripts are submitted with numerous singular/plural errors and the only advice I can give is to read every single sentence and then find the verb and decide whether it is singular or plural. It is not difficult. You just have to spend some time on it and then you will see it easily if it should be "was or were" or "has or have" or "is or are" and so on. Check it carefully since it is really irritating for the editorial office to get a paper where this is not fixed.

What is the error: "Melatonin levels was higher in men compared with women"

(it should be "were" in stead of "was")

Another point where at least foreigners like me will sometimes have problems is when writing the possessive form of nouns, where to put the apostrophe and where to put the "s". The key question is whether the noun is singular or plural, because in singular the apostrophe should come before the "s" and in plural it comes after the "s". It is actually not so difficult as long as you can distinguish between singular and plural. An example could be "one month's patients" and "four months' patients".

What is the error: "All NSAID's are ulcerogenic"

(It should be the simple plural form "NSAIDs", not the possessive form "NSAIS's")

The next thing is about the general use of abbreviations. This is a bad habit I must say for many writers, because if you use abbreviations you will slow down the speed of reading for the reader and this may sometimes be so annoying so the reader will leave you. He or she will skip your paper and read something else. Therefor be careful not to use too many abbreviations and especially do not use abbreviations that are not standard. Only use abbreviations that are fully accepted like for instance a CT-scan or MR-scan or something like that because this is part of the normal medical language and actually not anymore considered to be abbreviations in the sense of medical writing, so you are not obliged to spell them out first time they appear in the text. Be careful with abbreviations and keep it to an absolute minimum. If you have to use abbreviations you should also remember that all abbreviations should of course be spelled out the first time that they appear and your legends for tables and figures are considered unique areas of the text so the full spelling of the abbreviation should be repeated in the legends for tables and legends for figures as well as in the main text itself.

Another common confusion is how to abbreviate liter and milliliter. The most common way to do it is liter=L and milliliter=ml. You may find different methods in the literature, but it is important that you at least keep it consistent throughout the paper. I would suggest that you use L and ml, since these are most commonly used.

What is the error: "Two l of alcohol per person corresponding to 2,000 mL"

(Liter should be L and milliliter should be ml)

These were just some examples that you may benefit from and it is certainly not a comprehensive grammar lesson. Good luck with medical writing - be careful and check your text thoroughly because it has to be as perfect as you can do it. If you are not a native English speaker then you may benefit from sending your manuscript to a professional before you submit it to a journal. There are many options for this on the Internet and some of them are quite cheap and they will find the most obvious grammar and spelling errors. I will not recommend this for everybody but if you know that you have a weak spot here, then maybe it would be a good idea.

Closing

I sincerely hope that you have enjoyed this book and that you have picked up a few tricks for scientific writing.

The most important take home message is probably that you should use the exact same technique every time you write a scientific paper. If you stick to exactly the same outline build every time, then this will not be something that you have to worry about. You can switch on the autopilot, and that will make it a lot easier for you. Actually, this will by itself also help you overcome some of the writer's block that all are experiencing to some extent.

Writer's block is not a problem only for the young scientists; it may be a major problem even for the most experienced authors. The best way to overcome writer's block is probably to have strict habits for the writing process, and one of the key elements here is to build the research paper with a tight template every time you write a paper. Of course the templates differ depending on the type of paper, but use the same every time and then you have already won a little victory in the battle against writer's block.

The key to effective and successful scientific writing is to make the papers easy to read and easy to write, and you are already a large step into this process by using the strict templates and writing tips from this book. I therefore hope that you will benefit from the information in the book.

Notes

contact

www.biomedicalpublishing.com

www.ingramcontent.com/pod-product-compliance
Lightning Source LLC
Chambersburg PA
CBHW071822200526
45169CB00018B/702